The Recover Series

OPTIMIZE YOUR GUT

A Comprehensive Guide to Gut Health and Healing

DR. INDIGO VASQUEZ, DNM

ISBN: 979-8-8831-2860-7

A thank you is not enough to express the gratitude I have for those who have always told me that I am capable.

To my daughter Sofia, my husband, TJ, my mentor, AJ, Mom and Dad and many, many more.

You told me I could, so I did. Thank you.

Contents

❧❧❧

Foreword

Brandon Beckrich, Iron Rails Training Facility

AS A NUTRITIONIST, a personal trainer for twenty-plus years, and a functional medicine practitioner, I see so much human misery. And not just in the mentally ill, but also in the "normal," "healthy" population.

I also see the same unhappiness in the high-functioning, relatively successful people I work with within my own field. Quite often, the pain and misery are unnecessary and finally end when the people take charge of their beliefs, feelings, and actions, in order to modify the process of their lives.

Dr. Indie has routinely impacted lives for the better, mine included. She's a brilliant human with a heart worth her weight in gold, which she reveals to each and every patient she sees.

Brandon Beckrich, Nutritionist and Mindset Coach
Owner, Iron Rails Training Facility
Iron Rebel-Sponsored Athlete

ൠൠൠ

Foreword

A.J. Mihrzad, Online SuperCoach

DR. INDIE VASQUEZ is the catalyst you need to optimize your health at the highest level!

This book is so profound in its principles, especially after reading it while personally being coached by Dr. Indie to help heal a multitude of health problems, including my gut health. I urged her to write a book and was happy to work with her in starting it, completing it and now getting it published.

Dr. Indie has made major shifts in the health of her patients (including me) and it is by these exact strategies that you will make profound shifts in your gut health along with your overall well-being.

Dr. Indie has a gift of healing life-long ailments that doctors, medications and other health professionals are unable to solve. When I became sick, tired and had serious problems assimilating my foods, I personally saw many doctors, healers and "gut experts" but was not getting any better.

Then after following the protocol outlined in this book, it helped to heal my gut issues, optimized my digestion and most importantly she helped to improve my business productivity, energy and overall vitality! This is why I am even more honored that she chose me to write this foreword.

Dr. Indie is a loving, powerful woman who changes many lives and a Godsend to many like me to have suffered from long term health issues that seemed to be unsolvable. This book will be one of many that she writes and I know that it will change your life.

Being a fitness professional with 20 years of experience, a nutritionist, and an inductee into the personal training hall of fame, I've read hundreds of books about human anatomy, psychology, physiology, and science behind our delicate digestive system. I can honestly say that this is one of the most complete and comprehensive books when it comes to gut health and naturally healing our digestion with proven strategies.

Optimize Your Gut seriously gets my highest recommendation

With Love,

AJ Mihrzad

Author, *The MIND-BODY Solution: Train Your Brain for Permanent Weight Loss*
Founder, OnlineSupercoach.com

Introduction

My Story

THE BEST AND MOST compassionate healers tend to have experienced significant pain and suffering in their lifetime. It is thought in some indigenous cultures, that those who suffer the most, and those who have shown adversity in that suffering, are to be chosen as the tribe's healer. I think of this often when I look back at all of the health adversity I have had to overcome, to get to where I am today. I like to think that my suffering was a prerequisite, and requirement, so that I may be the best possible healer to those who come to me for guidance. After all, how can one offer advice for something that he or she has not also experienced? This perspective makes me grateful for it all.

Growing up, I was always sick. I was exhausted, in exceptional pain, suffering with gut issues, depression, anxiety, weight issues, absolutely freezing cold at all times. I had a hard time learning, remembering, thinking straight. Jeez!

I thought I was crazy and I definitely felt like I was dying.

My parents did their best for me, and although they showed concerns with the medical providers, we were told that I was fine. I should eat less and exercise more. Something you might have also heard.

I spent decades like this.

Once I became a Mother, the frustration of this invisible illness just became more frustrating. I had no energy to be the best Mother I knew I was. I had little patience, and could barely get through a day without needing significant time to recover. Everything was so challenging to complete. Life seemed so heavy and the guilt of having this illness and not being able to be the absolute best Mother, was excruciating. My daughter deserved better. I still have to work through this uncomfortable emotion to this day.

Because of my constant health concerns, and my deep desire to show my daughter the best version of myself, I naturally fell in love with an obsessive curiosity towards anything that could possibly help me heal.

Then, I finally met The One! The one practitioner who *finally* listened to me, who heard me, who told me that she could help me. She took the time needed to help me and because of her compassion and love for advocating for patients, she saved my life! I want everyone to have the opportunity to feel as heard and as hopeful as she made me feel.

This led me into a 15+ year study in nutrition therapy, natural medicine, and bioenergetic medicine.

These healing modalities have allowed me to finally overcome and optimize my body and mind. These healing techniques have allowed me to thrive, be present with my daughter, while also giving every patient I work with, 100% of me.

I wrote this book for those who feel unheard and frustrated with their health and want a straightforward, effective, and sustainable protocol that WILL help you feel better!

Have you struggled with your health? Have you been told that you're getting older and that, of course, you would be fatigued because of this? Have you been passed from Doctor to Doctor? Does this sound familiar to you?

If it does - you are in the right place, reading the right book!

I wrote this book for those who feel that they are not able to afford a fancy healing protocol with a fancy practitioner!

I wrote this book because I believe everyone should have access to safe and effective information that will help them reach their wellness goals.

Let's do this!

How To Use This Book

You can think of this book as a roadmap to better health. It should give a clear understanding on the how's and why's to gut health (and ultimately optimal health in general). We will take a deep dive into understanding how your gut influences health, biochemistry, physical disease, mental disease, and more.

We will also see more clearly the delineation between genetic influences and environmental influences and your health. Though- it is not always clear which has more influence on your health, it is very clear that both factors play a major role in deciding disease progression.

This roadmap will give you basic (but powerful) tools, in helping you reach your goals (hopefully that goal is optimal health).

Chances are, if you are reading this book, you are looking to advocate for yourself. This is fantastic news to me!

Let's get to the good stuff...

Chapter One

Understanding Your Gut

The Importance of Gut Health and the Gut-Body Connection

GUT HEALTH IS important for overall well-being and plays a crucial role in maintaining optimal mental and physical health. Here are some key reasons why gut health is so important!

* **Digestion and nutrient absorption:**

The gut (primarily the small intestine) is responsible for breaking down food and converting it into energy. A healthy gut ensures efficient digestion and nutrient absorption, which is essential for providing the body the energy and resources it needs to function optimally. Without gut health, you are unlikely to have good health!

* **Immune system support:**

Did you know? The gut houses a significant proportion of the body's immune system. A well-balanced gut microbiome (the community of microorganisms in the gut), helps regulate the immune system, protecting you against pathogens and other harmful bacteria. Do you tend to get colds every year? *Well* - it could be your gut environment! *How cool is that?* A strong gut barrier also protects against harmful bacteria from entering into the bloodstream. This is how many autoimmune diseases start, and even chronic allergies! Those allergies may not be so "seasonal" after-all.

* **Mental Health:**

The gut-brain connection (often called the gut-brain axis), is a bidirectional communication system between the gut and the brain. Emerging research suggests that the gut microbiome can influence mood, behavior, and even mental health conditions like anxiety and depression. A balanced gut can literally alleviate you from anxiety! *How cool is that?* With the decline of nutrients in our soul, and the chronic consumption of highly processed foods, *it is no wonder we are currently experiencing a mental health crisis.*

* **Weight Management:**

The gut microbiome can impact weight regulation and metabolism. Certain gut bacteria are associated with obesity, while others are linked with leanness! This means that you can alter your gut microbiome in such a way, to help you lose weight. *How cool is that?* A healthy gut can help you lose weight and ultimately keep it off.

* **Detoxification:**

The gut helps eliminate toxins and waste products from the body. A healthy gut, with an optimal functioning digestive system, is essential for effective detoxification. This means you are having at least *ONE* bowel movement per day. It is never normal to go more than one day without having a bowel movement.

The Important Role of the Microbiota

The microbiota refers to the diverse community of microorganisms, including bacteria, viruses, fungi, archaea, and single-celled organisms, that reside within and on the body. Our microbiota is mostly found in the intestinal tract but also exists in various other parts of the body, including your skin, oral cavity, and respiratory tract.

The role of the microbiota is vast and intricate, influencing several aspects of your health status. This includes your mental health, development, and general overall well-being. Protecting and optimizing the gut microbiome is the secret weapon to all aspects of health!

The Gut-Brain Axis

The gut-brain connection (often called the gut-brain axis), is a bidirectional communication system (you are going to hear this term often), between the gut and its microbiota with the brain and the central nervous system. This axis involves a complex interplay of neural, hormonal, and immune pathways. Whoa! This sounds kind of important right? Let's dive deeper into this, because it is very important to what we are about to accomplish with your gut healing program.

✓ Neurological Communication

The enteric nervous system (ENS), often referred to as "the second brain", is a network of neurons lining the gut. It can operate independently but also communicates with the central nervous system (CNS), through various nerves. Signals are transmitted between the gut and the brain via the vagus nerve, connecting the brain stem - to the abdomen. (More on the importance of this and how it relates to your self-care regimen in a later chapter).

✓ Hormonal Communication

The hormonal communication between the gut-brain axis is an amazingly complex system (also a bidirectional communication system), and plays a major role in hormone health. In my practice, I focus a lot on female hormone health, and our first step to all healing protocols, always begins in assessing the patient's gut health. I cannot get a woman's hormones in a balanced and comfortable place, without her having a well-functioning digestive system! This is also true in men's health. Because of this, we will dive deep into exactly how your hormones and your digestive health interact.

Let's talk about the various hormones and their role in overall health...

Enteroendocrine cells

The gut contains specialized cells called enteroendocrine cells. These cells are scattered throughout the intestinal tract, from the stomach to the small and large intestine. They are capable of sensing the presence of nutrients, as well as the physical and chemical conditions of the gut.

Enteroendocrine cells release various hormones into the bloodstream, in response to specific stimuli. Some of the most important gut hormones involved in gut-brain communication are:

Ghrelin: Ghrelin is often referred to as the "hunger hormone". It is primarily produced in the stomach and stimulates appetite. Ghrelin levels rise before meals and fall after eating.

Cholecystokinin (CCK): CCK is released in the response to the presence of fat and protein in the small intestine. It helps regulate digestion and reduces food intake by signaling to the brain that you are full.

Peptide YY (PYY): PYY is released by the ileum and colon in response to nutrients. It plays a role in reducing appetite by signaling satiety to the brain.

Glucagon-like peptide-1 (GLP-1): GLP-1 is secreted in the small intestine in response to the presence of food. It enhances insulin secretion and reduces appetite.

Leptin: Although primarily produced by adipose (fat) tissue, leptin also plays a role in gut-brain communication by regulating appetite. Leptin levels rise as fat stores increase, sending signals to the brain that you are full and reducing appetite.

Immunological Communication

The gut is a central player in the function of the body's immune system, and hormones (such as cortisol), a stress hormone, can modulate the immune response. Chronic stress, for instance, can lead to elevated cortisol levels, which (if left unchecked), can drive inflammation and lead to an imbalance in the gut microbiota.

Yes- one stressful event (even a short bout of anger), can alter your gut microbiome unfavorably. Cortisol plays a crucial role in the body's healing system though and is not the villain like it is portrayed. (The important role of cortisol can have its own book, so we will leave that for another conversation).

If left unchecked as mentioned, cortisol can potentially trigger an inappropriate immune response and potentially lead to an autoimmune disease.

Microbiota Influence

The gut-microbiota plays a significant role in metabolizing hormones, particularly estrogen. These microorganisms can either promote the excretion of estrogen or reabsorb it, affecting hormone levels in the body. An imbalance in the gut microbiota can lead to estrogen dominance, which is associated with various health issues, including hormonal imbalances and even an increased risk in estrogen fueled cancers.

Effects of Health and Well-being

Health and well-being can have a significant impact on gut health, and the relationship between the two is complex. The gut, which includes the stomach and intestines, plays a crucial role in digestion, nutrient absorption, and immune function. Let's talk about this in greater detail because it is crucial to optimal gut health, there is no way around it.

Chronic stress can affect the gut through the gut-brain access through a bidirectional communication system between the central nervous system and the enteric nervous system (the gut's own nervous system).

Did you know the gut has its own nervous system? Cool right? Stress can also lead to changes in gut motility, meaning you just cannot seem to have a daily BM no matter how much water you drink, or how much fiber you eat. This is largely due to being in "fight-or-flight."

Stress can even contribute or directly cause gut permeability issues (leaky gut), as well as drive irritable bowel syndrome.

For the reasons listed above, this protocol found in this book expresses and encourages, taking rest seriously. Self-care is a required component to healing, and it speaks a greater volume to your goal of optimizing your health than any supplement can.

❧❧❧

Chapter Two

Signs of an Unhealthy Gut

AN UNHEALTHY GUT can present in many different ways. Let's take our first self-assessment. Check the box for each symptom that you experience.

Self-Assessment for Gut Health

(Mark all that apply)

☐ I struggle with chronic constipation (less than one BM daily) or diarrhea

☐ I tend to feel gassy and/or bloated often (more than 3x/week)

☐ I struggle with persistent or recurrent discomfort in the abdominal area

☐ I experience heartburn or acid reflux

☐ I tend to have several food sensitivities or I struggle to digest certain foods

☐ I see undigested food in my stools

☐ I am concerned or feel that I have food allergies

☐ I tend to feel chronically fatigued or I get tired after eating certain foods

☐ I experience acne or skin irritation like eczema

☐ I tend to catch colds or get sick often/easily

☐ I struggle with bad breath and/or body odor

Now total your checked boxes, giving yourself one point for each box. If you scored:

0-3 points: Fantastic! It sounds like you are not struggling with food related symptoms. Your nutrition may be in a pretty good place, but maybe it could be a bit better (and that is why you are here, reading this book). Follow along and see where you might be able to improve!

>3 points: There is a good chance you may have food sensitivities or may be experiencing nutrient deficiencies (that lead to other symptoms). This book will help you gain the knowledge to help you empower yourself to find the root cause. Follow the

"Heal Your Gut" protocol as best as you can, paying close attention to how you feel when you have removed foods, as well as symptoms you experience when reintroducing foods.

The Link between Gut and Chronic Disease

Did you know that many chronic diseases are directly linked to poor gut health? Understanding these connections is crucial because we as consumers can make better informed choices when it comes to what we put in our body. Let's take a look at some common *(but not normal)*, and familiar diseases that are driven heavily by poor gut health.

Have you ever been told that you have IBS-D or IBS-C? Well, chronic inflammation in the intestinal tract can cause severe imbalances in your gut microbiota and is oftentimes the root issue. Even Ulcerative Colitis and Crohn's disease are commonly affected by a poor gut microbiome diversity.

Research also suggests a link between gut dysbiosis, and insulin resistance, playing a key role in the development of Type 2 Diabetes.

❧❧❧

Chapter Three

Causes of Gut Imbalances

Poor Diet

DID YOU KNOW? A poor diet (one rich in processed foods and beverages, and light on high quality meats, fruits, and veggies), can significantly impact not only your gut health, but your long-term health. We have already talked in detail about how the gut microbiome plays a crucial role in the body as a whole, but let's dive deeper into how diet specifically is important for maintaining good gut health.

A diet low in fiber and high in processed foods, sugars, and unhealthy fats can disrupt the balance of the gut microbiota. Fiber is beneficial for nourishing beneficial gut bacteria, and a lack of good gut bacteria can lead to an overgrowth of harmful bacteria.

Chronic inflammation can impair the integrity of the gut barrier, allowing harmful substances to leak into the blood steam. This is commonly known as leaky gut syndrome. Common yes - but normal - NO!

A poor diet can increase the risk of gastrointestinal disorders, irritable bowel syndrome (IBS-D or IBS-C), and inflammatory bowel disease (IBD). These are disorders that have a deeper root cause. A diagnosis of IBS or IBD is more often a *symptom*, and not the true issue.

Sleep

Poor sleep habits and quality can disrupt the circadian rhythms of the gut, impacting the gut's ability to function optimally. Disrupted sleep patterns may affect the diversity of the gut bacteria and contribute to issues like leaky gut syndrome and inflammation. (More on this later in the book).

Exercise

Regular physical activity has been shown to have a positive impact on gut health. Exercise can promote the growth of beneficial gut bacteria and improve gut motility. Sedentary behavior, however, may negatively affect gut health.

Hydration

Staying hydrated is imperative for maintaining gut health. Water is essential for digestion and helps prevent constipation. It is also important to note that proper hydration is more than just drinking water. A balanced mineral status in water, and including salt and electrolytes to your drinking water improves overall hydration. Did you know - you can actually force dehydration by taking too much water that contains too little minerals? More on this later...

Smoking and alcohol

Smoking cigarettes and consuming alcohol can negatively affect gut health. Smoking can damage the gut lining and drinking alcohol can disrupt the balance of gut bacteria. It will be very challenging to heal a gut, if the patient is not willing to also give up alcohol. Alcohol acts as a sanitizer in the gut. It destroys bacteria, but the issue is that it does not discriminate between friendly versus unfriendly bacteria. This poses a huge problem when you are attempting to heal the gut, and gut healing requires a balanced gut microbiome. For this reason, I strongly encourage patients to discontinue all alcohol consumption when working on healing, ideally, for the long term.

Mental health

Mental health and gut health are (once again), interconnected in a bidirectional manner. Research in recent years has shed light on the strong relationship between the two, and it is an area of growing interest in both medical and scientific communities. This subject is too complex to dive deep into, in this book, but let us take a look at the most significant factors that cause gut imbalance when considering mental health.

The most common (but not normal) factor when considering both mental health and gut health, is inflammation. Inflammation is a common feature in many mental health disorders and gastrointestinal conditions. The gut is a significant source of systemic inflammation, and an imbalanced gut microbiome can contribute to chronic inflammation. This chronic inflammation may play a role in the development or exacerbation of mental health conditions. Disruptions in the gut microbiome have been linked to conditions like depression, anxiety, panic disorders, and many other conditions.

Emerging research suggests that interventions aimed at improving gut health, such as probiotics, prebiotics, and dietary modifications, may have a positive impact on mental health conditions.

Additionally, addressing mental health issues through therapy, certain herbs and supplements, and stress reduction techniques, can have a beneficial impact on gut health.

Medications and Antibiotics

Medications and antibiotics can have various effects on the health of the gut, both positive and negative. The gut is home to a complex community of microorganisms (which we talk about repeatedly in this book), and plays a crucial role in maintaining overall health.

Here is how medications and antibiotics can affect the gut:

✓ **Antibiotics:**

Antibiotics are designed to kill or inhibit the growth of bacteria, and they do not discriminate between harmful and beneficial bacteria. This can disrupt the balance of the gut microbiota, leading to several potential side effects. Let's take a look at what those potential side effects look like.

Dysbiosis: Antibiotics can lead to a condition called dysbiosis, where there is an imbalance in the gut microbiota. This may result in an overgrowth of harmful bacteria and a decrease in beneficial bacteria.

Gastrointestinal symptoms: Taking antibiotics can oftentimes cause loose stools, constipation, nausea, bloating and other discomforts. These are primarily caused by an imbalance in the gut microbiota.

Increased susceptibility to infections: A disrupted gut microbiota can leave the body more vulnerable to opportunistic infections. It is unfortunately common to experience recurring infections after taking antibiotics.

Long-term effects: Some studies suggest that repeated or prolonged antibiotic use may be associated with an increased risk of conditions like irritable bowel syndrome (IBS) and inflammatory bowel disease (IBD).

✓ **Other Medications:**

Various medications can affect the gut in different ways, depending on their mechanism of action. Here are some examples:

Non-steroidal anti-inflammatory drugs (NSAIDS): These drugs, such as Ibuprofen and aspirin, can irritate the gastrointestinal lining, potentially leading to ulcers and bleeding in the gut.

Proton Pump Inhibitors (PPIs): These drugs, often used to treat heartburn and acid reflux, can alter the PH of the stomach and reduce the production of stomach acid, which may affect the gut's ability to digest and absorb nutrients. This can also allow undesirable pathogens to enter the GI tract, causing distress and even recurring UTI infections. There are gut friendlier ways to address heartburn and acid reflux without these drugs.

Corticosteroids: These medications can increase the risk of infections, as they suppress the immune system.

Immunosuppressants: Drugs that affect the immune system, such as those used in organ transplant patients or autoimmune diseases, can increase the risk of gut infections, and drive GI distress overall.

Positive Effects

Some medications, such as probiotics, are designed to support gut health. Probiotics are beneficial bacteria that can be taken as supplements or found in certain foods. I generally recommend getting probiotics from foods, as there are several studies that show taking probiotics supplementally can increase the risk of small intestinal bacterial overgrowth (SIBO). I use specific probiotics for very specific GI symptoms, and never use them as a general wellness product.

It is also important to remember that antibiotics and other medications have varying effects from person to person. When using antibiotics, it is essential to follow your healthcare provider's guidance while also being informed about the potential side-effects. In some cases, probiotics or dietary recommendations may be made to protect or restore gut health after treatment.

ଔଔଔ

Chapter Four

The Gut-Healing Quick-View

(If you just want to get started NOW)

Using Food as Medicine

NUTRITION PLAYS A crucial role in maintaining gut health and overall well-being. Remember - gut health = optimal health. You cannot find healing without it!

Foods to Avoid for the First Six Weeks of Your Gut Healing Protocol

- ✓ Highly processed foods
- ✓ Sugary foods and drinks
- ✓ Fried and fatty foods
- ✓ Conventional raised meats (grass-fed is safe)

- ✓ Dairy products
- ✓ Gluten-containing foods
- ✓ Alcohol
- ✓ Egg yolks
- ✓ Seeds/Nuts
- ✓ Nightshade vegetables
- ✓ Soy
- ✓ Grains
- ✓ Corn
- ✓ All refined flours and sugars

Sneaky Ingredients to Avoid

Some ingredients sound harmless but are in fact not ideal for your gut or your general well-being. Do not be fooled by these ingredients found on food labels.

- **Sugar**

Agave nectar

Brown rice syrup

Organic cane sugar

Ethyl Maltol

Dextrose

Fructose

Fruit juice concentrate

Barley malt (syrup)

Cane juice (evaporated cane juice)

Beet Sugar

Carob syrup

- **Oils**

Canola oil

Vegetable oil

Soybean oil

Palm oil

Cottonseed oil

Grapeseed oil

Corn oil

Sunflower oil (used in moderation and never heated)

Safflower oil (used in moderation and never heated)

Sesame oil (used in moderation and never heated)

Peanut oil (used in moderation and never heated)

- **Added Flavors**

Natural Flavors

Monosodium glutamate

High-fructose corn syrup

Aspartame

Sucralose

Saccharin

Acesulfame Potassium

Artificial Flavor

Yeast extract

- **Added Colors**

All added colors should be avoided. Red 40, yellow 5, and yellow 6, are known to drive behavioral problems in children and adults.

- **Emulsifiers**

Carboxymethyl cellulose (CMC)

Polysorbate 80 (P80)

Carrageenan

Polyglycerols

Xanthan gum

Soy Lecithin

- **Preservatives**

Sodium nitrite

Sodium benzoate

Potassium bromate

BHA

BHT

Propyl Gallate

Sulphites

It is important to note: individual tolerance to these foods can vary, and some people may be able to tolerate certain items on this list without issues.

Foods to Focus on For the First Six Weeks of Your Gut Healing Protocol (even better: long-term)

These foods are:

* Prebiotic and probiotic rich foods

* Resistant starches

* Foods that feed commensal bacteria

- **Probiotic Rich Products**

Probiotic-rich foods are important for the gut because they contain live microorganisms, primarily beneficial bacteria, that provide several health benefits when consumed regularly. Let's dive more into this topic, because it is important!

Some of my favorite probiotic rich foods are…

- ✓ Kimchi
- ✓ Sauerkraut
- ✓ Kombucha
- ✓ Kefir (dairy)
- ✓ Yogurt (dairy if tolerated or a coconut milk alternative)

Beneficial functions of probiotic rich foods are…

- **Maintaining gut microbiota balance:**

Probiotics help to balance the composition of bacteria in the gut. The human gut is home to trillions of bacteria, both good and bad. Does knowing you are full of bacteria make you feel weird?

Consuming probiotic rich foods can help ensure that the delicate balance of bacteria is in favor of the beneficial bacteria, which is essential for digestive health.

- **Supports optimal digestion:**

Foods rich in probiotics aid in the breakdown of food and the absorption of nutrients in the digestive tract. They can help alleviate symptoms of digestive disorders like loose stools, constipation, IBS (irritable bowel syndrome), and IBD (irritable bowel disease).

- **Boosts immunity:**

A significant portion of the body's immune system resides in the gut. Choosing to consume foods rich in probiotics can help support immune function by enhancing the gut barrier, which prevents harmful bacteria from entering the bloodstream and causing infections. They also stimulate the production of antibodies and promote the activity of immune cells.

- **Reduces Inflammation:**

Some strains of probiotics have anti-inflammatory properties, which can help alleviate inflammation in the gut and throughout the body. Chronic inflammation is linked to various health problems, including autoimmune diseases and metabolic disorders.

- **Enhances Mental Health:**

Emerging research suggests that the gut-brain axis, the bidirectional communication between the brain and the gut, plays a crucial role in mental health. Probiotic rich foods may help improve mood and reduce symptoms of anxiety and depression by modulating the gut microbiota and influencing neurotransmitter production.

- **Supports Overall Health:**

In addition to supporting specific benefits for gut health, probiotic rich foods can also support weight management, improve skin appearance, and reduce the risk of certain chronic diseases.

Notice how I did not mention or encourage specific probiotic supplementation outside of food forms. This is because supplementing with a probiotic product should be done with strategy. Data is suggesting that taking oral probiotic supplements for general wellness purposes, has been shown to drive SIBO (small intestine bacterial overgrowth), a very challenging issue to correct.

It is best to always implement foods first, before supplements in general, and if you decide to use a supplement, choose a spore based option (these are most friendly to your gut microbiome and less likely to cause SIBO).

The Superheros of the Gut Healing Protocol are Resistant Starches

Resistant starches serve as prebiotics, meaning they are indigestible by human enzymes in the small intestine, but can be fermented by beneficial bacteria in the colon. This fermentation process produces short-chain fatty acids (SCFAs) such as acetate, propionate, and butyrate, which are essential for colon health and have been associated with reduced inflammation and improved gut barrier function. These foods should be consumed daily!

Some of my favorite resistant starch foods are:

* Cooked and *cooled* potato (of all forms)

* Cooked and *cooled* wild and black rice

* Cooked and *cooled* black beans

* Real sourdough bread made from a starter and not commercial yeast

I leverage resistant starch foods heavily in a gut healing protocol, because of how powerful they are in balancing the gut microbiome. Not only do these foods improve gut microbiome, resistant starches also:

* Regulate blood sugar

* Support weight loss and can even reduce the occurrence of weight loss resistance

* Reduce colon cancer risk

I encourage you to try to make a sourdough starter at home! Let me know how you do...

Foods that Feed Commensal Bacteria

Commensal bacteria are a diverse community of trillions of bacteria that inhabit your intestinal tract. They play an important role in defending against pathogens, by acting on the host's immune system to induce protective responses which in turn reduce your chances of getting sick. They aid in digestion - synthesizing essential nutrients and also support certain metabolic functions, making them important to focus on, if your goal is weight loss. With that reason, implementing foods that feed commensal bacteria is vital to general gut health.

Some of my favorite foods that feed commensal bacteria are:

* Slightly green bananas (not too green though because it can cause digestive upset)

* Apples with the skin left on

* Blackberries, raspberries, blueberries

- ✻ Grapefruit (use caution when on certain prescription medications)

- ✻ Broccoli, kale, spinach, carrot

- ✻ Walnuts, chia seeds, flaxseeds

ⓒⓇⓒⓇⓒⓇ

Chapter Five

Healing Your Gut Through Lifestyle

Stress Management

SELF-CARE AND RELAXATION (or finding rest and recovery), are very important for gut health. Why? Because your nervous system directly affects your digestive system! When you experience traumatic events, chronic and acute stress, and other things like poor sleep quality, your nervous system will be stuck in what is called "sympathetic dominance", or "fight-or-flight".

Why is this not ideal?

Because when your body is in this state, it preserves energy and focuses it on keeping your organs as optimized as possible. This means that the gut will slow down.

This is why implementing self-care and relaxation techniques are an important part of your gut healing protocol.

Let's do a quick self-assessment to determine if stress may be affecting your gut health. Check all that apply!

☐ I tend to struggle with anxiety

☐ I often feel down or depressed

☐ I struggle with feeling tired often, or I would call myself fatigued in general

☐ I often feel bloated or gassy, or experience loose stools or constipation

☐ I feel like I have several food sensitivities

☐ I get headaches often (more than once a week)

☐ I struggle with high blood pressure

☐ My libido is generally low

☐ I have mood swings or I feel irritable in general

☐ I struggle to concentrate

☐ I often do not feel rested when I wake up

☐ I do not get at least 7 hours of sleep per night

☐ I feel like I can not lose weight, even if I eat well and exercise

❧❧❧

How did you do? If you checked more than three of these, stress is very likely driving some of the gut distress! Now, the key here is to know what to do, to help your nervous system feel safe again.

Now is a great time to talk about them...

Sleep

Ah sleep, the magic elixir of life! Sleep and stress management are closely intertwined. Adequate and high quality sleep is crucial for emotional and physical well-being, cognitive function, and overall resilience when dealing with stress. Of course, this translates into how well your gut functions as well!

To effectively manage stress, protect sleep over getting those dishes done, or that laundry put away! By the way- the laundry and dishes will never be done... so... let's focus on what we can control (which is protecting your recovery - sleep)!

A few things you can do to get better sleep are:

- ✓ Take time to watch the sunrise in the morning. Exposing your eyes to the morning light is crucial for a healthy circadian rhythm

- ✓ Avoid electronics one hour before bed

- ✓ Use blue-light blockers before bed (and really any time you are exposed to blue light)

- ✓ Create a consistent bedtime routine (and protect it)

- ✓ Only use caffeine two hours after waking up, then discontinuing caffeine consumption 6 hours prior to bedtime.

- ✓ Avoid alcohol in general but especially before bed

- ✓ Avoid late night eating (ideally discontinue food three hours prior to bedtime)

Exercise

Engaging in regular physical activity can promote relaxation and decrease muscle tension. Activities like yoga, stretching, or deep breathing activities, can also help your body recover from a tendency for higher cortisol, and promote a "rest-and-digest" state of being. The key is finding activities that you *actually* enjoy, and set a realistic goal for yourself if it has been awhile since you hit your sport or activity.

If you have been sedentary for a bit, please take it slow.

Exercise both creates and uses cortisol. If you are someone who is often anxious or has signs of excess cortisol, you may want to avoid or limit high intensity workouts to twice per week. Low and moderate intensity exercise can be very helpful in controlling cortisol levels.

Hydration

Staying hydrated is crucial for overall health- most people know that! But WHY? Let's talk about it.

- **Digestion and Nutrient Absorption:**

Adequate water intake is essential for the digestion of food. Water helps break down larger molecules into smaller and more easily absorbed components. This process allows nutrients to be absorbed more efficiently through the walls of the intestines and into the bloodstream.

- **Constipation Prevention:**

Insufficient water intake can lead to constipation. Water softens the stool, making it easier to pass through the intestines. Without enough water, stools can be hard and difficult to move, driving poor bowel movement frequency. That's not very comfortable!

- **Mucous production:**

The lining of the GI tract produces mucus to protect the tissues and aid in the movement of food. Water helps maintain the production of this protective mucous layer, preventing irritation and damage to the GI tract.

If we do not get enough water, chronic dehydration may contribute to the development of certain gastrointestinal disorders, such as peptic ulcers and gastritis. Maintaining adequate hydration helps prevent these conditions and supports overall gut health.

It is important to note that individual water needs vary based on factors such as age, weight, activity level, and climate. As a general guideline, aiming for 50% of your body weight in ounces of water per day is often recommended, but individual needs may vary. It is always good to listen to your body and adjust your water intake accordingly.

❧❧❧

Chapter Six

Detoxification

DETOXIFYING THE GUT is an important practice, especially in our current environment! In today's world, toxins are everywhere. They are in our food, water, the air we breath, household cleaners, cosmetics, and much more.

Unfortunately, we cannot avoid toxins completely, so the best possible chance at pushing towards optimal health is to focus on being consistent in practicing healthy lifestyle techniques to enhance our body's detox abilities. No, I am not talking about doing a juice cleanse or committing to some expensive gut detox kit (which is generally not good for you anyways). I am talking about gentle, sustainable, and generally very affordable self-care methods to help improve your ability to detoxify.

Toxins and Gut Health

Here are the main players in your body's detoxification system:

Digestive tract: Helps expel toxins and excess waste through your stool

Lymphatic system: Known as "the garbage men" for your body. Your lymphatic system transports white blood cells that fight infection via the lymph, a fluid that circulates throughout your body.

Kidneys: Filters toxins and then excretes them through your urine.

Liver: Filters toxins from your blood and helps eliminate harmful pathogens, heavy metals, excess hormones (especially estrogen), and chemicals.

Lungs: Converts toxins into CO_2 which then gets exhaled.

Skin: Your largest eliminatory organ and your body's first line of defense. Your skin helps you detox via your sweat.

Simple ways to support detox include:

Drink plenty of water: This keeps your bowels moving and helps the kidneys do their job.

Aim to drink approximately 2 liters of filtered spring water each day.

Manage stress: Living in "fight or flight" mode impairs detox. So practice daily stress relief. Yoga, meditation, journaling, and listening to calm music are all good options.

Deep breathing: Helps your lungs filter toxins and promotes relaxation. Try some box breathing or breath of fire. You can find great guided breathwork exercises on Youtube.com.

Exercise: Staying active improves circulation and keeps your bowels and lymph moving. I recommend at least 30 minutes of gentle movement, like walking or cycling, every day. Strength training is also very important for general health. Aim for at least three strength-training days per week.

Need more potent detox support? Whether you are on a heavy metal cleanse, candida detox protocol, or just wanting to upgrade your gut health, the following six methods will help.

1. Sauna or sauna blanket

One of the easiest ways to rid your body of toxins is to sweat them out. As an added bonus, sauna stimulates the parasympathetic nervous system (aka "rest and digest mode"), which is crucial for effective detox. You can use a sauna at a nearby gym or spa or consider investing in a sauna blanket.

2. Dry brushing

This Ayurvedic technique improves blood flow, exfoliates the skin, moves the lymph, and may even reduce the appearance of cellulite. All you need is a natural bristle brush. Start at the feet and brush in long sweeping motions towards the heart. Dry brushing is best done before showering or bathing.

3. Rebounding

Believe it or not, jumping on a mini trampoline can help you detox. The up-and-down motion stimulates the lymphatic system to help flush out toxins. As an added bonus, it may help reduce cellulite too. Try rebounding for 3-5 minutes at a time, working up to 15 minutes a day.

4. Detox baths

Epsom salts contain magnesium, a mineral that helps your muscles relax, and is critical for detox. Soaking in an Epsom Salt bath helps flush out harmful toxins while easing stress and promoting relaxation. Simply add 2 cups of Epsom salts to a warm bath and feel your stress melt away.

5. Coffee enemas

While it may sound weird, this method involves injecting warm coffee into your rectum and colon and then retaining it for around 15 minutes. Coffee enemas cleanse the liver, relieve constipation, reduce inflammation, promote immunity, and boost your energy. They also flush out harmful yeast, bacteria, parasites, and heavy metals.

6. Castor oil packs

This folk remedy promotes liver detoxification and stimulates the lymphatic system. To make a castor oil pack, soak a piece of wool or cotton flannel in castor oil and place it on the right side of your abdomen. Then apply a heating pad for around 30-45 minutes.

7. Tongue scraping

What goes on in your mouth affects your entire body. Scraping your tongue first thing in the morning helps you remove harmful bacteria, toxins, and dead cells. The result? Better breath, enhanced sense of taste, and improved oral health. When choosing a tongue scraper, opt for stainless steel or copper product.

❧❧❧

Chapter Seven

Heal Your Gut

Functional Approach to Whole-Body Wellness

THE FOLLOWING IS your Four-Step Guide to Improve the Health of Your Gut for Optimal Wellness, the "Four-R Program," inspired by Dr. Jeffrey Bland!

For best results, follow each step in order. The next step will often overlap with the previous.

The Four-R Program

As per Dr. Jeffery Bland

Step 1. Remove and Repair (Weeks 1-6): The first week starts with no dairy, no grains or gluten, and no soy containing products. Reduce consumption of toxins and inflammatory foods (as well as foods that you are possibly sensitive to). These foods and other chemical ingredients were listed in chapter four.

Step 2. Replace (Weeks 1-6): Give your liver a deep breath of fresh air by implementing foods specifically designed to help improve detoxification and overall gut health. Some supplements are recommended, but consuming whole foods and proper hydration is most important. Supplements can support the process but will not keep you in long term health. Focus on whole foods and use organic produce and grass-fed meats if you are able to. Implement the resistant starches and foods that feed commensal bacteria.

Step 3. Reinoculate (Weeks 1-6): Bring in specific probiotics and prebiotics to help recalibrate the gut microbiome. Probiotics are the healthy gut bacteria found in fermented foods while prebiotics are foods that feed the probiotics. Probiotic supplements should always be used with caution and under the supervision of a practitioner familiar with using probiotics, as supplementing outside of necessity can drive undesirable imbalances. These foods were listed in chapter four.

Step 4. Repair (Week 7 and on): Start to reintroduce foods that you have eliminated, with the most nutrient dense foods first to fully replenish the body and return to a natural way of eating. This is a great time to implement your food and symptom tracking journal. Take 3-5 days eating the new food in at least two meals per day. If you have a reaction, remove the food and wait one week to re-introduce the next food group. Gluten is not necessary to add back into your diet and can be helpful to remove long term, though some choose to add this back in small quantities.

Reminder: a **balanced diet** should come before any supplement routine.

❧❧❧

Supplements

Listed below are my favorite go-to supplements to support a gut-healing protocol. These are generalized recommendations and you may require more strategic support based on your unique needs.

Always speak to your functional medicine provider before starting any supplement regimen.

- **Zinc picolinate 15mg**

Zinc is fabulous for gut health, because it is responsible for repairing the cells that line the intestinal tract and helps maintain a healthy mucosal lining. Zinc can also reduce inflammation and free-radical damage, protect against the ever-so-common H. pylori bug, and can help balance the gut microbiome.

Zinc in the picolinate form is shown to be highly bioavailable, as well as much gentler on your stomach. Many zinc products (especially oxide), can cause nausea.

- **Fermented Cod Liver Oil 2,000-3,000mg in divided doses**

I recommend a fermented form of fish oil, because many brands (even the well respected ones), tend to use heat in their manufacturing process, which damages the fragile medicine in the oil, causing oxidation and of course - potentially driving inflammation in the body. Enough with inflammation, am I right?

- **L-glutamine powder 5g**

L-glutamine is an amino acid that supports gastrointestinal health by repairing the gut wall and can help ease the symptoms of leaky gut (as well as protect against it). L-glutamine is also an energy source for intestinal and immune cells, which help protect against harmful bacteria or toxins.

This product is best taken on an empty stomach, either 30 minutes before your first meal of the day, or two hours after your last meal of the day.

- **Biologically Active Methyl B-complex**

Did you know? B vitamins play a crucial role in supporting optimal microbiome diversity, while also suppressing the growth of less favorable bacteria! This is a lesser known (but very important fact).

Many B vitamins are produced using synthetic ingredients. This can be frustrating to your body, as we generally do not recognize (at the cellular level) synthetic versions of any vitamin or mineral. A biologically active B complex is made from fruits and veggies, which is *naturally* friendlier to the metabolism especially if you have an MTHFR genetic polymorphism.

Quick tip: It is estimated that 40% of the population carries this gene mutation! It can drive GI distress, anxiety, fatigue, mood imbalances and more. I would consider getting tested if you have not already. Your primary care physician can run this test for you, or you are always welcome to order a test kit for yourself!

☙☙☙

Chapter Eight

Tracking your Progress

NOW, IT IS TIME TO bring everything together and start getting to work! A few last items to consider before diving into your protocol...

Keeping a Gut-health Journal

Keeping a gut health journal can be beneficial for a number of reasons, especially if you are dealing with gastrointestinal issues or trying to improve your health. Identifying food triggers is very important for truly finding your specific food sensitivities. Otherwise, it can be challenging to figure out where your digestive discomfort, bloating, and other symptoms are coming from. Gut health journals are also beneficial for:

* Tracking symptoms

* Assessing progress

* Providing data for health care providers

* Logging how stress and lifestyle affects your gut health

* Keeps you accountable and focused

* Gives you the unique and personal approach to healing you need

To keep a gut healing journal effectively, it is important to be consistent, honest, and thorough in your recording. Include details about what you eat and drink, portion sizes, symptom severity and duration, and any other relevant factors like stress levels or medication use. This information can be a valuable resource for both you and your healthcare team when working towards better gut health.

How to Monitor your Symptoms

Monitoring your gut health is crucial for understanding and managing your digestive well-being. Here is a simple guide to help you effectively monitor your gut health:

- **Keep a food diary (we just discussed this in detail in the previous chapter)**

Record what you eat and drink daily, including portion sizes and ingredients. This can help identify potential triggers for digestive issues.

Note any unusual or uncomfortable symptoms during or after meals.

- **Track symptoms**

Record specific digestive symptoms, such as bloating, gas, loose stool, constipation, stomach cramps and heartburn.

Note the frequency and severity of these symptoms, and any potential patterns or triggers.

Be as detailed as possible in your descriptions.

If you are interested in using my food log, please email me, and I will send you the document! There are many ways to do this, however. You can find printable .pdfs, books on Amazon that are dedicated to food tracking, or simply use a notebook.

- **Monitor bowel movements**

Pay attention to the frequency, consistency, and color of your bowel movements. The Bristol Stool Scale can help you classify stool types.

Note any changes in your normal bowel habits.

- **Identify potential triggers**

Try to identify any specific foods or beverages that seem to worsen or alleviate your gut symptoms.

Consider lifestyle factors, stress factors, stress levels, sleep patterns, and physical activity as potential triggers and contributors to your gut health.

- **Record medications and supplements**

Keep track of any medications or dietary supplements you are taking, as they can affect your gut health.

Document any changes in medication or supplement usage and their effects.

- **Keep a stress diary**

Emotional health can have a significant impact on gut health. Consider keeping a stress diary to monitor stressful events and your body's physical responses to stress.

- **Measure progress**

Over time, assess whether changes in your diet, lifestyle, or medication are positively (or negatively), affecting your gut health. Make adjustments as needed.

Remember that everyone's gut health is unique, and it may take time to pinpoint the causes of digestive issues. Keeping a detailed record of your symptoms and daily habits can provide valuable insights and help healthcare professionals make accurate diagnoses and recommendations for managing your gut health.

Piecing it all Together

Committing to long-term gut healing is crucial, as we have learned that the gut plays a major role in your overall well-being. Having a qualified health practitioner on your side can make a world of a difference and provides a valuable asset on your quest for health and healing.

My hope for you, in writing this book, is to provide empowering and powerful knowledge, so that you can feel comfortable and ready to take control of your health and healing experience.

Let's take you off of the roller-coaster ride of symptoms you may be experiencing. Let's help you find balance and optimal health.

I want to give you something to support your first steps to optimizing your gut health!

I am offering you a free 4-week gut healing program as a gift for successfully completing this book. This program will give you a more in-depth protocol to help put into action the strategies found in this book.

To receive your free 4-week gut healing program, simply email me at:

thedenvernaturopath@gmail.com

I will send a .pdf containing exclusive additional information, not found in this text, with the hope that it will continue to inspire you to keep working towards optimization.

You may also connect with me on the Instagram social media platform at:

@Dr.IndigoVasquez

In health and healing,

Indigo Vasquez

Testimonials

Testimonial #1: Alyssa Butor, Denver, CO

Before I met Indie I struggled with severe stomach issues for probably 5-6 years. I went to multiple Doctors and was told the reason for my discomfort is that "I'm aging" (I was 26 years old at the time.) I was told "My stomach may just not work as well as it used to", or my personal favorite "I don't see anything wrong with you."

I found Dr. Indigo and said - enough is enough- my stomach deserves better! I finally made an appointment and within 15 minutes she could tell my stomach acid was low and was contributing to 85% of my problems. ARE YOU SERIOUS?! 15 minutes to find out what took multiple Doctor's visits and years of dead-end answers. Low stomach acid? Wow. Dr. Indie put me on the right regimen (for my unique needs), and within 3 days I was feeling like a new woman. I am forever grateful for finding Dr. Indigo and her methods of healing.

Testimony #2: Ashley Steinberg, Denver, CO

I discovered Indie at a pivotal moment, a perfect storm of challenges. After nearly two years of unsuccessful attempts to conceive, my husband and I faced the fact that we were going to need fertility help. I was not excited for the conventional path and was looking for anything else we could do before heading to a fertility clinic. A career transition put me under extreme stress to the point I was losing my hair. Additionally, I was fed up with a decade-long struggle against abnormal symptoms—persistent fatigue and year-round congestion. Coupled with a family medical history laden with conditions I hoped to avoid—such as stroke, heart attack, and cancer—I sought a proactive, natural approach to healing.

It was during this time a friend suggested I see Indie, and I promptly scheduled an appointment. Quickly, she pinpointed a potential low-functioning thyroid and identified an overloaded stress response system. Indie recommended targeted supplementation, dietary adjustments (excluding dairy, gluten, and sugar), and tapping therapy.

Within two months, I felt like a brand-new person. It was clear to me and my husband that her protocol was effective. Further hormone and mineral testing provided a comprehensive view of my needs, unveiling a gene mutation and significant mineral imbalances. Indie personalized a protocol, encompassing supplementation, dietary changes, detox routines, breathwork, and other therapies, addressing my specific requirements.

Although it took two years to uncover root cause answers, each appointment marked progress in various aspects. Together, Indie and I successfully alleviated my stress response systems, reduced inflammation, tackled extreme fatigue, balanced hormones, and unearthed a crucial gene mutation. A decade of working with traditional doctors yielded no results, as they never delved beyond surface-level "normal" lab results. In contrast, Indie diligently addressed and improved every aspect within two years.

Her responsiveness to questions, comprehensive guidance, and meticulous follow-up notes surpassed any previous experiences. Indie's affordability and consideration of costs in supplement recommendations and additional testing exemplify her dedication and heart. She is the only person who truly heard and believed me, treating me holistically rather than as a list of symptoms. We were so impressed with Indie and her practice that my husband decided to see her as well. Words cannot adequately express the profound positive impact Indie has had on our lives. We are eternally grateful for her knowledge, influence, honesty, kindness, and unwavering passion for facilitating our healing journey. We now understand that healing is not only possible but also that we don't need to tolerate symptoms just because we've grown accustomed to them.

Testimony #3: Lexie Maitland, Florida

I reached out to Indie in Jan of 2023 after battling some awful symptoms that I wrote off for so long. My thyroid was extremely out of whack but most importantly, and where Indie was a GODSEND, was that she dug deeper and identified that the root of my thyroid issues were chronic stress and gut related. This was something that my previous practitioner had failed to mention. This also explains why I had been put on thyroid medication by my prior practitioner and had seen absolutely no changes to my bloodwork. Before Indie, I felt STUCK. And hopeless, to say the least.

When I finally took action and reached out to Indie, she made me feel heard and cared for. Her calm and soothing nature really put me at ease in our initial consultation. I also really appreciated how she walked me through everything so thoroughly and explained the nature of what we were going to do regarding my healing protocol. I felt so at peace and cared for after our first consult. It only took one meeting with Indie for me to gain complete trust.

Flash forward to almost a YEAR later and a YEAR of working with Indie and I have not only learned SO much, but I feel like the athlete I knew I had the potential to feel like. My symptoms from Jan 2023 have done a COMPLETE 180 since starting with Indie AND I was able to undergo a successful prep in the midst of this past year, under her guidance with my health supplement regimen.

I could not recommend Indie enough and as an athlete in the extreme sport of bodybuilding, it is so amazing to know that I have someone who always has my health in the forefront of her mind AND who cares for me as a person and athlete. Indie is truly one of a kind and I don't say this lightly, but she is perhaps one of the best things to happen to me in 2023.

Testimonial #3, Charleigh C., Denver, CO

Dr. Indie has helped me greatly along my journey with Complex Regional Pain Syndrome (CRPS). My CRPS is a chronic nerve condition that specialists and doctors approach mainly with medication and drugs such as gabapentin. Gabapentin is known to induce over seventy negative side effects.

My mom hoped to avoid this type of treatment, given the adverse outcomes. When we heard of Dr. Indie through a friend, it seemed she was exactly what we were looking for. Dr. Indie was so welcoming and answered as many of our questions as she could. She is always willing to adjust our treatment plan or schedule to fit our needs, which is so comforting. Just two months into treatment with Dr. Indie, I began to notice small improvements.

With my CRPS, it was difficult to compete in wrestling, soccer, and other sports that I love. Now, more than a year later, I am able to play my favorite sports with little interference from my nerve pain. We have changed my treatment plan a few times over the course of our work together, and I am 100% confident the only reason I'm feeling as good as I am is because of Dr. Indie's recommendations, knowledge, and guidance. My family will be forever grateful for her and what she has done for my quality of life!

Testimony #4: Cliff Weidel, San Antonio, TX

Dr. Indigo Vasquez helped me discover first, what was ailing me, and second what I could do about it. I'm a Senior now and over the years I have damaged my gut with injuries, infections, and poor diet. I started feeling poorly, having lots of reflux and general sluggishness.

I had no idea what was going on but Dr. Indie sure did. She was great at listening to me and started me on the road to recover slowly by making some changes to my diet and offering some suggestions with some gut supplementation. She is very caring and knowledgeable.

I had no idea how beneficial natural medicine can be. I learned a little bit about the huge gap between traditional western medicine and natural medicine. There are so many things that can be done to improve one's health just by slowing down and taking control of what and how you do things. Dr. Indie is a competent professional expert and she coached me back to better health. Today I am feeling much better as I continue my journey and discovery on how to take charge of my life. I know there are skeptical people out there because I was one of them. But, not any more.

ଓଓଓଓ

About the Author

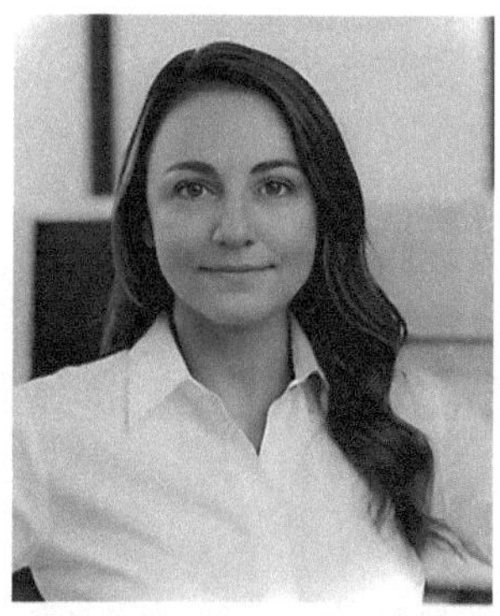

INDIGO VASQUEZ, DNM (Dr. Indie) holds doctoral degrees in Natural Medicine, Bioenergetic Medicine, and Sacred Medicine. She works to help patients revitalize their hormone health through comprehensive healing protocols, including gut healing and nervous system optimization.

Dr. Indie also holds diplomas in both Psycho-Physiological Bioenergetic Allopathic Medicine and Herbalism and Energy Psychotherapy. She has also completed an NASM certification in personal training, a certification in Auriculomedicine, and a certification in Bioenergetic Medicine.

Dr. Indie's whole-body approach to healing offers patients new avenues to achieve their wellness goals.